DR. BARBARA 7-DAY GUT CLEANSE

Transform your gut health in just 7-days with dr. Barbara's expert cleanse: discover digestive renewal, vitality and wellness with proven strategies for a healthier life

Miguel Sofia

COPYRIGHT © 2023

CHAPTER ONE

Introduction to Dr. Barbara's Gut Cleanse: Understanding the Importance of Gut Health in Overall Well-being

The human gut, often referred to as the gastrointestinal (GI) tract, is a marvel of biological engineering, comprising a complex ecosystem of microorganisms, enzymes, and cells working in harmony to digest food, absorb nutrients, and maintain overall health. In recent years, scientific research has illuminated the profound impact of gut health on various aspects of well-being, from physical health to mental acuity and even emotional stability. As our understanding of the gut microbiome deepens, so too does our appreciation for the critical role it plays in maintaining equilibrium within the body.

The Gut Microbiome: A Diverse Ecosystem

At the heart of gut health lies the microbiome, a vast and diverse community of microorganisms that inhabit the digestive tract. These microorganisms, which include bacteria, viruses, fungi, and archaea, collectively weigh as much as three pounds and outnumber human cells by a factor of ten. Far from being mere passengers in the gut, these microbes actively contribute to various physiological processes, such as nutrient metabolism, immune function, and even mood regulation.

The composition of the gut microbiome is influenced by numerous factors, including genetics, diet, lifestyle, and environmental exposures. While certain species of bacteria are considered beneficial and promote health, others can be harmful if allowed to proliferate unchecked. Maintaining a balanced microbiome is thus crucial for optimal gut function and overall well-being.

The Gut-Brain Axis: Bridging Body and Mind

One of the most fascinating discoveries in gut research is the existence of the gut-brain axis, a bidirectional communication network linking the digestive system with the central nervous system. This intricate relationship allows for constant signaling between the gut and the brain, influencing everything from appetite and mood to cognitive function and stress response.

The gut microbiome plays a pivotal role in modulating this communication network, producing neurotransmitters, such as serotonin and dopamine, that are essential for mood regulation and emotional stability. Disruptions in the gut-brain axis have been implicated in various neurological and psychiatric disorders, including depression, anxiety, and autism spectrum disorders.

The Impact of Modern Lifestyles on Gut Health

In recent decades, shifts in dietary patterns, widespread antibiotic use, and increased exposure to environmental toxins have taken a toll on gut health worldwide. Highly processed foods, high in sugar, unhealthy fats, and artificial additives, have been shown to disrupt the delicate balance of the gut microbiome, promoting the growth of pathogenic bacteria and inflammation.

Moreover, the overuse of antibiotics, while instrumental in combating bacterial infections, can indiscriminately wipe out beneficial gut bacteria, leaving the microbiome vulnerable to colonization by harmful pathogens. Chronic stress, another hallmark of modern life, has also been shown to dysregulate gut function, leading to gastrointestinal disorders and systemic inflammation.

The Role of Gut Cleansing in Restoring Balance

Recognizing the importance of gut health in maintaining overall well-being, many health practitioners have turned to gut cleansing protocols as a means of restoring balance to the microbiome and promoting digestive wellness. Dr. Barbara's Gut Cleanse is one such protocol designed to support the body's natural detoxification pathways and replenish beneficial gut bacteria.

At the core of Dr. Barbara's Gut Cleanse is a holistic approach that combines dietary modifications, nutritional supplements, and lifestyle interventions to optimize gut function and enhance overall health. By eliminating inflammatory foods, such as gluten, dairy, and processed sugars, and incorporating nutrient-dense whole foods rich in fiber, antioxidants, and essential nutrients, the cleanse aims to nourish the gut microbiome and reduce intestinal inflammation.

The Benefits of Gut Cleansing

Proponents of gut cleansing tout a myriad of potential benefits, including improved digestion, enhanced nutrient absorption, increased energy levels, and better immune function. By removing toxins and supporting the growth of beneficial gut bacteria, a cleanse may also alleviate symptoms associated with gastrointestinal disorders, such as bloating, gas, constipation, and diarrhea.

Moreover, emerging research suggests that gut cleansing may have far-reaching effects beyond digestive health, influencing systemic inflammation, metabolic function, and even mental well-being. By restoring balance to the gut microbiome and promoting a healthy gut-brain axis, a cleanse may help mitigate symptoms of anxiety, depression, and other mood disorders.

Conclusion: Empowering Health through Gut Cleansing

In conclusion, the importance of gut health in maintaining overall well-being cannot be overstated. From its central role in digestion and nutrient absorption to its influence on mood, cognition, and immune function, the gut plays a multifaceted role in human health. Understanding the intricate interplay between the gut microbiome, the gut-brain axis, and various lifestyle factors is essential for optimizing gut function and promoting longevity.

Dr. Barbara's Gut Cleanse offers a comprehensive approach to gut health, harnessing the power of dietary modifications, nutritional supplementation, and lifestyle interventions to support the body's natural detoxification processes and promote digestive wellness. By restoring balance to the gut microbiome and nurturing the gut-brain axis, a cleanse may hold the key to unlocking vibrant health and vitality.

CHAPTER TWO

The Gut Microbiota: Exploring the Role of Beneficial Bacteria in Digestive Health

The gut microbiota, a complex ecosystem of microorganisms residing within the gastrointestinal tract, plays a pivotal role in maintaining digestive health and overall well-being. Comprising trillions of bacteria, fungi, viruses, and other microorganisms, the gut microbiota forms a dynamic community that interacts with the host organism in myriad ways. In this exploration, we delve into the fascinating world of beneficial bacteria and their profound impact on digestive function, nutrient metabolism, and immune regulation.

The Diversity of Gut Microorganisms

The human gut is home to a vast array of microorganisms, collectively known as the gut microbiota. This microbial community is incredibly diverse, with thousands of different species coexisting within the confines of the digestive tract. Among these microorganisms, bacteria are the most abundant and well-studied, comprising hundreds of species belonging to various phyla, including Firmicutes, Bacteroidetes, Actinobacteria, and Proteobacteria.

Despite their small size, gut bacteria exert a tremendous influence on host physiology, contributing to essential functions such as nutrient metabolism, energy extraction, and immune modulation. Moreover, recent research has revealed the intricate interplay between gut bacteria and human health, highlighting the importance of maintaining a balanced and diverse microbiota for optimal well-being.

The Role of Beneficial Bacteria

Within the vast landscape of the gut microbiota, certain bacteria are considered beneficial due to their positive effects on digestive health and overall physiology. These beneficial bacteria, often referred to as probiotics, exert a range of beneficial effects, including:

1. **Digestive Enzyme Production**: Beneficial bacteria produce enzymes that aid in the breakdown and digestion of complex carbohydrates, proteins, and fats, facilitating nutrient absorption and promoting digestive comfort.

2. **Fermentation of Dietary Fiber**: Some beneficial bacteria specialize in fermenting dietary fiber, a process that produces short-chain fatty acids (SCFAs) such as acetate, propionate, and butyrate. SCFAs serve as an energy source for colonocytes (cells lining the colon) and play a crucial role in maintaining gut barrier integrity and modulating immune function.

3. **Competitive Exclusion of Pathogens**: Beneficial bacteria compete with pathogenic microorganisms for space and

resources within the gut, thereby reducing the colonization and proliferation of harmful bacteria. This competitive exclusion mechanism helps to maintain a healthy microbial balance and protect against gastrointestinal infections.

4. **Immune Modulation**: Beneficial bacteria interact with the host immune system, stimulating the production of anti-inflammatory cytokines and promoting immune tolerance. By modulating immune function, probiotic bacteria help to prevent inflammatory disorders and maintain gut homeostasis.

Examples of Beneficial Bacteria

Several genera of bacteria are renowned for their beneficial effects on digestive health and overall well-being. Among the most well-studied probiotic species are:

1. **Lactobacillus**: Lactobacillus species are lactic acid-producing bacteria found in various fermented foods, such as yogurt, kefir, and sauerkraut. These bacteria are known for their ability to colonize the gastrointestinal tract, inhibit the growth of pathogenic bacteria, and modulate immune function.

2. **Bifidobacterium**: Bifidobacteria are another group of beneficial bacteria commonly found in the human gut. These bacteria play a crucial role in fermenting dietary fiber and producing SCFAs, which contribute to gut health and

immune regulation. Bifidobacterium species are often included in probiotic supplements due to their beneficial effects on digestive function.

3. **Saccharomyces boulardii**: While not a bacterial species, Saccharomyces boulardii is a beneficial yeast that has been extensively studied for its probiotic properties. This yeast is known for its ability to support digestive health, alleviate symptoms of gastrointestinal disorders, and prevent antibiotic-associated diarrhea.

Maintaining Gut Microbiota Balance

Maintaining a balanced and diverse gut microbiota is essential for promoting digestive health and overall well-being. Several factors influence the composition and diversity of the gut microbiota, including diet, lifestyle, medications, and environmental exposures. To support the growth of beneficial bacteria and maintain gut microbiota balance, individuals can:

1. **Consume a Diverse Diet**: Eating a varied diet rich in fruits, vegetables, whole grains, and fermented foods provides essential nutrients and promotes microbial diversity within the gut.

2. **Limit Intake of Processed Foods**: Highly processed foods high in sugar, unhealthy fats, and artificial additives can disrupt the gut microbiota and promote the growth of

pathogenic bacteria. Limiting consumption of these foods supports gut health and overall well-being.

3. **Take Probiotic Supplements**: Probiotic supplements containing beneficial bacteria, such as Lactobacillus and Bifidobacterium species, can help restore microbial balance in individuals with dysbiosis or digestive disorders.

4. **Avoid Overuse of Antibiotics**: While antibiotics are essential for treating bacterial infections, their overuse can disrupt the gut microbiota and lead to dysbiosis. Whenever possible, use antibiotics judiciously and consider probiotic supplementation to mitigate their effects on gut health.

5. **Manage Stress**: Chronic stress can impact gut function and alter the composition of the gut microbiota. Practicing stress-reduction techniques such as mindfulness, meditation, and regular exercise can help support gut health and promote microbial balance.

Conclusion

In conclusion, the gut microbiota plays a critical role in maintaining digestive health and overall well-being. Beneficial bacteria within the gut microbiota contribute to essential functions such as nutrient metabolism, immune modulation, and pathogen exclusion. By promoting the growth of beneficial bacteria through dietary modifications, probiotic supplementation, and lifestyle interventions, individuals can support gut health and optimize microbial balance. A deeper understanding of the role of beneficial bacteria in digestive health offers insights into novel therapeutic approaches for gastrointestinal disorders and underscores the importance of nurturing the gut microbiota for lifelong wellness.

CHAPTER THREE

Gut Health and Disease: Understanding How Imbalances in the Gut Microbiome Contribute to Illness

The human gut microbiome, a complex ecosystem of microorganisms residing within the gastrointestinal tract, plays a crucial role in maintaining overall health and well-being. However, disruptions in the delicate balance of the gut microbiome, known as dysbiosis, have been implicated in the pathogenesis of various diseases and disorders. In this exploration, we delve into the intricate relationship between gut health and disease, examining how imbalances in the gut microbiome contribute to illness across a spectrum of conditions.

Dysbiosis: A Disruption of Gut Microbiome Balance

Dysbiosis refers to an imbalance in the composition and diversity of the gut microbiome, characterized by alterations in the relative abundance of beneficial and pathogenic microorganisms. This disruption of microbial equilibrium can arise from various factors, including dietary patterns, lifestyle choices, medications, and environmental exposures. Dysbiosis has been linked to numerous health conditions, ranging from gastrointestinal disorders to systemic inflammatory diseases.

Gut Microbiome and Gastrointestinal Disorders

Dysbiosis of the gut microbiome is strongly associated with the pathogenesis of gastrointestinal disorders, including inflammatory bowel diseases (IBD), such as Crohn's disease and ulcerative colitis, as well as irritable bowel syndrome (IBS). In individuals with IBD, dysbiosis is characterized by a reduction in microbial diversity and alterations in the abundance of specific bacterial taxa, such as increased levels of Proteobacteria and decreased levels of Firmicutes.

These microbial changes can lead to intestinal inflammation, epithelial barrier dysfunction, and immune dysregulation, contributing to the chronic inflammatory processes observed in IBD. Similarly, dysbiosis has been implicated in the pathogenesis of IBS, with alterations in gut microbiota composition and function contributing to visceral hypersensitivity, altered gut motility, and gastrointestinal symptoms such as abdominal pain, bloating, and diarrhea.

Gut Microbiome and Metabolic Disorders

Emerging research has highlighted the role of the gut microbiome in the development of metabolic disorders, including obesity, type 2 diabetes, and non-alcoholic fatty liver disease (NAFLD). Dysbiosis of the gut microbiome has been associated with obesity-related metabolic dysfunction, characterized by alterations in energy harvest, adipose tissue inflammation, and insulin resistance.

Specifically, an imbalance in the ratio of Firmicutes to Bacteroidetes bacteria, known as the "obese microbiota phenotype," has been observed in individuals with obesity and metabolic syndrome. This dysbiotic microbiota profile is thought to promote energy extraction from the diet and contribute to adiposity and metabolic dysregulation.

In addition to obesity, dysbiosis of the gut microbiome has been implicated in the pathogenesis of type 2 diabetes, with alterations in gut microbiota composition and function influencing glucose metabolism, insulin sensitivity, and systemic inflammation. Moreover, dysbiosis has been linked to the progression of NAFLD, a common liver condition characterized by hepatic steatosis and inflammation, suggesting a potential role for gut microbiome-targeted interventions in managing metabolic disorders.

Gut Microbiome and Immune-Mediated Diseases

The gut microbiome plays a critical role in modulating immune function and tolerance, and dysbiosis has been implicated in the pathogenesis of immune-mediated diseases, including autoimmune disorders and allergic conditions. In autoimmune diseases such as rheumatoid arthritis, systemic lupus erythematosus, and multiple sclerosis, dysbiosis of the gut microbiome may contribute to immune dysregulation and the breakdown of self-tolerance.

Alterations in gut microbiota composition and function have also been linked to allergic diseases, including asthma, allergic rhinitis, and atopic dermatitis. Dysbiosis of the gut microbiome during infancy has been associated with an increased risk of allergic sensitization and the development of allergic disorders later in life, highlighting the importance of early-life microbial colonization in immune development and disease susceptibility.

Conclusion

In conclusion, the gut microbiome plays a pivotal role in maintaining health and homeostasis throughout the body. Dysbiosis, or imbalances in the gut microbiome, can contribute to the pathogenesis of a wide range of diseases and disorders, including gastrointestinal disorders, metabolic diseases, and immune-mediated conditions. Understanding the intricate relationship between gut health and disease offers insights into novel therapeutic strategies for managing and preventing these conditions, highlighting the potential of gut microbiome-targeted interventions in promoting health and well-being. Further research into the mechanisms underlying gut microbiome dysbiosis and its impact on disease pathogenesis is needed to develop more effective treatments and interventions aimed at restoring microbial balance and improving patient outcomes.

CHAPTER FOUR

Dr. Barbara's Approach to Gut Cleansing: Principles of Herbal Therapy and Nutritional Support

Dr. Barbara's gut cleansing protocol represents a holistic approach to digestive wellness, drawing upon principles of herbal therapy and nutritional support to promote optimal gut health and overall well-being. Grounded in the belief that nature provides powerful remedies for restoring balance to the body, Dr. Barbara's approach combines the therapeutic properties of herbs with targeted nutritional interventions to support the body's natural detoxification processes and nourish the gut microbiome.

Herbal Therapy: Harnessing the Healing Power of Plants

Herbal therapy, also known as botanical medicine or phytotherapy, has been used for centuries as a primary mode of healing in traditional medical systems worldwide. Herbs contain a myriad of bioactive compounds, including alkaloids, flavonoids, terpenes, and phenolic acids, which exert a range of pharmacological effects on the body. In the context of gut cleansing, certain herbs are prized for their ability to support digestive function, promote detoxification, and soothe gastrointestinal discomfort.

Principles of Herbal Therapy in Gut Cleansing

Dr. Barbara's gut cleansing protocol incorporates several key principles of herbal therapy to support digestive health and detoxification:

1. **Bitter Herbs for Digestive Stimulation**: Bitter herbs, such as dandelion root, gentian, and wormwood, are renowned for their ability to stimulate digestive secretions and promote optimal digestion. By enhancing gastric acid production, bile flow, and pancreatic enzyme release, bitter herbs help to improve nutrient absorption and alleviate symptoms of bloating, gas, and indigestion.

2. **Carminative Herbs for Gas Relief**: Carminative herbs, including fennel, peppermint, and ginger, possess anti-spasmodic and anti-inflammatory properties that help to relieve gas, bloating, and abdominal discomfort. These herbs relax the smooth muscles of the digestive tract, reduce intestinal spasms, and expel trapped gas, providing relief from digestive disturbances.

3. **Demulcent Herbs for Mucosal Protection**: Demulcent herbs, such as marshmallow root, slippery elm, and licorice, contain mucilaginous compounds that coat and soothe the mucous membranes of the gastrointestinal tract. These herbs form a protective barrier against gastric irritants, reduce

inflammation, and promote healing of the gut lining, making them valuable allies in gut cleansing protocols.

4. **Antimicrobial Herbs for Pathogen Clearance**: Certain herbs possess antimicrobial properties that can help eradicate pathogenic bacteria, fungi, and parasites from the gut. Herbs such as berberine-containing plants (e.g., goldenseal, Oregon grape), garlic, and oregano oil exhibit broad-spectrum antimicrobial activity and may be used to address dysbiosis and intestinal infections.

Nutritional Support: Nourishing the Gut Microbiome

In addition to herbal therapy, Dr. Barbara's gut cleansing protocol emphasizes the importance of nutritional support for nourishing the gut microbiome and promoting digestive wellness. A nutrient-dense diet rich in fiber, antioxidants, vitamins, and minerals provides essential building blocks for gut health and supports the growth of beneficial bacteria within the microbiome.

Principles of Nutritional Support in Gut Cleansing

Dr. Barbara's approach to nutritional support in gut cleansing encompasses the following principles:

1. **Fiber-Rich Foods for Microbiome Health**: Dietary fiber serves as a prebiotic substrate for beneficial bacteria in the

gut, promoting the growth of species such as Bifidobacteria and Lactobacillus. Consuming a variety of fiber-rich foods, including fruits, vegetables, whole grains, legumes, and nuts, helps to nourish the gut microbiome and support microbial diversity.

2. **Antioxidant-Rich Foods for Inflammation Control**: Antioxidants, found in abundance in colorful fruits and vegetables, help to neutralize free radicals and reduce oxidative stress in the body. By quenching inflammation, antioxidants support gut health and protect against oxidative damage to the gastrointestinal mucosa.

3. **Protein Sources for Tissue Repair**: Adequate protein intake is essential for tissue repair and maintenance of gut barrier integrity. Including high-quality protein sources such as lean meats, fish, poultry, eggs, dairy, and plant-based proteins in the diet provides amino acids necessary for healing and regeneration of the gut epithelium.

4. **Hydration for Digestive Function**: Proper hydration is essential for optimal digestive function and detoxification. Drinking an adequate amount of water throughout the day helps to maintain bowel regularity, support nutrient absorption, and facilitate the elimination of toxins from the body.

Conclusion

In conclusion, Dr. Barbara's approach to gut cleansing integrates principles of herbal therapy and nutritional support to promote digestive wellness and restore balance to the gut microbiome. By harnessing the healing power of herbs and providing essential nutrients for gut health, Dr. Barbara's protocol offers a comprehensive strategy for supporting optimal digestion, detoxification, and overall well-being. Incorporating herbal remedies and nutrient-rich foods into a holistic gut cleansing regimen can help individuals achieve lasting improvements in digestive health and experience the benefits of a revitalized microbiome.

CHAPTER FIVE

Preparing for the Cleanse: Guidelines for Pre-Cleanse Preparation and Transitioning to Gut-Cleansing Foods

Embarking on a gut cleanse can be a transformative journey towards improved digestive health and overall well-being. However, proper preparation is essential to ensure a smooth transition into the cleanse and optimize its effectiveness. In this guide, we'll explore key guidelines for pre-cleanse preparation and transitioning to gut-cleansing foods, setting the stage for a successful cleansing experience.

Pre-Cleanse Preparation: Setting the Foundation

Before diving into the cleanse, it's essential to lay the groundwork for success by preparing both physically and mentally. Here are some guidelines to consider during the pre-cleanse preparation phase:

1. **Assess Your Readiness**: Take stock of your current dietary habits, lifestyle factors, and health goals. Reflect on your reasons for undertaking the cleanse and set realistic expectations for the process.

2. **Consult with a Healthcare Professional**: If you have any underlying health conditions or concerns, consult with a

healthcare professional before starting the cleanse. They can provide personalized guidance and ensure that the cleanse is safe and appropriate for your individual needs.

3. **Gradually Reduce Intake of Stimulants**: To minimize potential withdrawal symptoms, gradually reduce your intake of stimulants such as caffeine, alcohol, and refined sugars in the days leading up to the cleanse. This can help ease the transition into a cleaner, more nourishing diet.

4. **Increase Hydration**: Hydration is key to supporting the body's natural detoxification processes. Start increasing your water intake in the days before the cleanse, aiming for at least 8-10 glasses of water per day. You can also incorporate hydrating foods such as fruits and vegetables into your diet.

5. **Stock Up on Cleansing Foods**: Take inventory of your pantry and refrigerator and stock up on gut-cleansing foods such as leafy greens, cruciferous vegetables, berries, nuts, seeds, whole grains, legumes, and lean proteins. Having these ingredients on hand will make it easier to stick to your cleanse plan.

Transitioning to Gut-Cleansing Foods: Gradual Changes for Long-Term Success

Transitioning to a gut-cleansing diet involves gradually eliminating processed foods, inflammatory ingredients, and potential allergens while increasing the intake of nutrient-dense, gut-supportive foods. Here's how to make the transition as smooth as possible:

1. **Focus on Whole Foods**: Prioritize whole, minimally processed foods in your diet, including plenty of fruits, vegetables, whole grains, legumes, nuts, seeds, and lean proteins. These foods are rich in fiber, antioxidants, vitamins, and minerals, which support gut health and overall well-being.

2. **Eliminate Common Triggers**: Identify and eliminate common dietary triggers that may exacerbate digestive issues, such as gluten, dairy, refined sugars, artificial additives, and processed foods. These substances can contribute to inflammation, dysbiosis, and gastrointestinal discomfort.

3. **Increase Fiber Intake**: Gradually increase your fiber intake by incorporating a variety of fiber-rich foods into your meals, such as leafy greens, cruciferous vegetables, berries, flaxseeds, chia seeds, and whole grains. Fiber supports digestive regularity, promotes satiety, and nourishes beneficial gut bacteria.

4. **Support Digestive Enzymes**: Include foods rich in digestive enzymes, such as pineapple (containing bromelain) and papaya (containing papain), to aid in the breakdown and digestion of macronutrients. Additionally, fermented foods

like sauerkraut, kimchi, kefir, and yogurt contain beneficial probiotics that support gut health.

5. **Stay Mindful of Portions**: Pay attention to portion sizes and listen to your body's hunger and fullness cues. Overeating, even with healthy foods, can strain the digestive system and lead to discomfort. Aim for balanced, satisfying meals that leave you feeling energized and nourished.

Conclusion

Preparing for a gut cleanse involves careful planning, mindful dietary choices, and gradual transitions to gut-cleansing foods. By laying the foundation for success during the pre-cleanse preparation phase and implementing gradual changes to your diet, you can support optimal digestive health and set yourself up for long-term wellness. Remember to listen to your body, stay hydrated, and seek support from healthcare professionals or nutrition experts if needed. With dedication and commitment, a gut cleanse can be a powerful catalyst for transformation and renewed vitality.

CHAPTER SIX

The 7-Day Gut Cleanse Protocol: Step-by-Step Instructions for Daily Herbal Supplements and Dietary Changes

Embarking on a 7-day gut cleanse can kickstart your journey towards improved digestive health and overall well-being. This protocol combines targeted herbal supplements with dietary changes to support detoxification, promote gut healing, and nourish beneficial gut bacteria. Follow these step-by-step instructions for a comprehensive cleanse experience.

Day 1: Preparation and Goal Setting

1. **Assess Readiness**: Take stock of your current dietary habits, lifestyle factors, and health goals. Reflect on your reasons for undertaking the cleanse and set realistic expectations for the process.

2. **Consult with a Healthcare Professional**: If you have any underlying health conditions or concerns, consult with a healthcare professional before starting the cleanse. They can provide personalized guidance and ensure that the cleanse is safe and appropriate for your individual needs.

3. **Stock Up on Supplies**: Purchase the necessary herbal supplements and gut-cleansing foods for the week ahead.

Ensure you have a variety of fruits, vegetables, whole grains, legumes, nuts, seeds, and lean proteins on hand.

Day 2-7: Daily Protocol

Morning Routine:

1. **Start Your Day with Lemon Water**: Upon waking, drink a glass of warm water with freshly squeezed lemon juice. This helps stimulate digestion, hydrate the body, and support detoxification.

2. **Take Herbal Supplements**: Follow the recommended dosage instructions for the herbal supplements included in the cleanse protocol. These may include digestive support herbs such as dandelion root, ginger, and licorice, as well as probiotics to replenish beneficial gut bacteria.

Breakfast:

1. **Enjoy a Gut-Cleansing Breakfast**: Choose a breakfast that includes gut-supportive foods such as overnight oats with berries, chia seeds, and almond milk, or a smoothie made with leafy greens, avocado, banana, and protein powder.

Mid-Morning Snack:

1. **Nourish with Nutrient-Dense Foods**: Snack on whole fruits, raw vegetables, or a small handful of nuts and seeds to keep energy levels stable and support gut health.

Lunch:

1. **Opt for Gut-Cleansing Lunch Options**: Enjoy a nourishing lunch featuring a colorful salad with leafy greens, cruciferous vegetables, avocado, and grilled chicken or tofu. Dress with olive oil and lemon juice for added flavor.

Afternoon Snack:

1. **Satisfy Hunger with Healthy Snacks**: Choose snacks that provide sustained energy and support digestive health, such as hummus with carrot sticks, Greek yogurt with berries, or a small serving of whole-grain crackers with almond butter.

Dinner:

1. **Finish the Day with a Light, Digestible Meal**: Prepare a balanced dinner consisting of lean protein, steamed vegetables, and a small portion of whole grains or legumes. Avoid heavy, processed foods that may burden the digestive system.

Evening Routine:

1. **Wind Down with Herbal Tea**: Before bed, enjoy a soothing cup of herbal tea such as chamomile, peppermint, or ginger. Herbal teas can help relax the body, promote restful sleep, and support digestion.

2. **Practice Relaxation Techniques**: Take time to unwind and de-stress before bed. Practice relaxation techniques such as deep breathing, gentle stretching, or meditation to promote relaxation and support overall well-being.

Additional Tips for Success:

1. **Stay Hydrated**: Drink plenty of water throughout the day to support detoxification and maintain hydration levels. Aim for at least 8-10 glasses of water per day, and hydrate with herbal teas, coconut water, and infused water for added flavor.

2. **Listen to Your Body**: Pay attention to how your body responds to the cleanse and make adjustments as needed. If you experience any discomfort or unusual symptoms, consult with a healthcare professional.

3. **Prioritize Sleep**: Aim for 7-9 hours of quality sleep each night to support detoxification, hormone balance, and overall health. Create a relaxing bedtime routine and optimize your sleep environment for restful slumber.

4. **Practice Mindful Eating**: Slow down and savor each bite during meals, paying attention to hunger and fullness cues. Chew food thoroughly, and avoid distractions such as TV or screens to promote mindful eating and digestion.

Conclusion

By following this 7-day gut cleanse protocol, you can support detoxification, promote gut healing, and nourish beneficial gut bacteria for improved digestive health and overall well-being. Remember to consult with a healthcare professional before starting any cleanse or dietary program, and listen to your body's needs throughout the process. With dedication and commitment, a gut cleanse can be a transformative experience towards renewed vitality and vitality.

CHAPTER SEVEN

Supporting Digestive Function: Identifying Key Herbs and Nutrients for Gut Healing and Repair

A healthy digestive system is essential for overall well-being, as it is responsible for breaking down food, absorbing nutrients, and eliminating waste. When the gut is compromised, it can lead to a range of digestive issues, including bloating, gas, indigestion, and more serious conditions like leaky gut syndrome and inflammatory bowel disease (IBD). Fortunately, certain herbs and nutrients have been shown to support digestive function and promote gut healing and repair. Let's explore some of these key herbs and nutrients:

1. Marshmallow Root (Althaea officinalis):

Properties: Marshmallow root contains mucilaginous compounds that coat and soothe the mucous membranes of the digestive tract, providing relief from inflammation and irritation. It also acts as a demulcent, helping to protect and heal the gut lining.

Benefits: Marshmallow root is beneficial for individuals with conditions such as gastritis, GERD (gastroesophageal reflux disease), and inflammatory bowel diseases like Crohn's disease and ulcerative colitis. It can help reduce inflammation, ease digestive discomfort, and support gut healing.

2. Slippery Elm Bark (Ulmus rubra):

Properties: Slippery elm bark is rich in mucilage, a gel-like substance that coats the digestive tract and provides a protective barrier against irritants. It also has anti-inflammatory and demulcent properties, making it useful for soothing and healing the gut lining.

Benefits: Slippery elm bark is commonly used to alleviate symptoms of conditions such as gastritis, ulcers, irritable bowel syndrome (IBS), and colitis. It can help reduce inflammation, soothe digestive discomfort, and promote healing of the gastrointestinal mucosa.

3. Chamomile (Matricaria chamomilla):

Properties: Chamomile is well-known for its calming and anti-inflammatory properties, making it beneficial for soothing digestive upset and reducing inflammation in the gut. It also acts as a carminative, helping to relieve gas and bloating.

Benefits: Chamomile is often used to alleviate symptoms of indigestion, bloating, cramping, and nausea. It can help relax the muscles of the digestive tract, ease tension, and promote overall digestive comfort.

4. Peppermint (Mentha piperita):

Properties: Peppermint contains menthol, a compound that has been shown to relax the muscles of the digestive tract and reduce symptoms of gastrointestinal distress. It also has anti-inflammatory and carminative properties, making it useful for soothing digestive discomfort.

Benefits: Peppermint is commonly used to alleviate symptoms of irritable bowel syndrome (IBS), including abdominal pain, bloating, and gas. It can help relax the muscles of the intestines, reduce spasms, and promote smoother digestion.

5. Licorice Root (Glycyrrhiza glabra):

Properties: Licorice root contains glycyrrhizin, a compound with anti-inflammatory and demulcent properties that can help soothe and heal the gut lining. It also has adaptogenic properties, helping to support overall digestive health and resilience.

Benefits: Licorice root is beneficial for individuals with conditions such as gastritis, ulcers, acid reflux, and leaky gut syndrome. It can help reduce inflammation, protect the gastrointestinal mucosa, and support the body's natural healing processes.

Key Nutrients for Gut Healing and Repair:

In addition to herbal remedies, certain nutrients play a crucial role in supporting digestive function and promoting gut healing and repair. These include:

1. **L-Glutamine:** An amino acid that serves as a primary fuel source for the cells lining the intestinal tract, supporting gut barrier function and promoting tissue repair.

2. **Zinc:** Essential for maintaining the integrity of the gut lining and supporting immune function in the digestive tract.

3. **Vitamin A:** Supports mucosal repair and regeneration in the digestive tract, helping to maintain a healthy gut lining.

4. **Omega-3 fatty acids:** Found in fish oil, flaxseed oil, and walnuts, omega-3 fatty acids have anti-inflammatory properties and support gut health by reducing inflammation in the digestive tract.

5. **Probiotics:** Beneficial bacteria that support a healthy balance of microorganisms in the gut, promoting digestion, nutrient absorption, and immune function.

Conclusion:

Incorporating key herbs and nutrients into your diet and supplement regimen can support digestive function, promote gut healing and repair, and alleviate symptoms of gastrointestinal distress. Marshmallow root, slippery elm bark, chamomile, peppermint, and licorice root are all valuable herbs with properties that soothe inflammation, protect the gut lining, and support overall digestive health. Additionally, nutrients such as L-glutamine, zinc, vitamin A, omega-3 fatty acids, and probiotics play essential roles in maintaining gut integrity and supporting optimal digestive function. Always consult with a healthcare professional before starting any new herbal or supplement regimen, especially if you have underlying health conditions or are taking medications.

CHAPTER EIGHT

DR. BARBARA RECIPES FOR GUT CLEANSE

1. **Lemon Ginger Detox Drink**

   - **Definition:** This drink helps to flush out toxins from the digestive system and promotes gut health.

   - **Ingredients:** Freshly squeezed lemon juice, grated ginger, water, honey (optional).

   - **How to Prepare:** Mix lemon juice and grated ginger in water. Add honey for sweetness if desired.

   - **How to Use:** Drink it first thing in the morning on an empty stomach.

   - **Dosage:** One glass daily.

   - **Side Effect:** May cause acidity in some individuals.

   - **Precaution:** Avoid if you have acid reflux issues.

2. **Green Smoothie**

   - **Definition:** A nutrient-dense smoothie that aids digestion and provides essential vitamins and minerals.

   - **Ingredients:** Spinach, kale, cucumber, green apple, celery, water or coconut water.

   - **How to Prepare:** Blend all ingredients until smooth.

- o **How to Use:** Consume as a breakfast or snack option.

- o **Dosage:** One serving per day.

- o **Side Effect:** None expected, but excessive consumption may lead to excess fiber intake.

- o **Precaution:** Monitor fiber intake if prone to digestive issues.

3. **Turmeric Detox Tea**

- o **Definition:** Turmeric is known for its anti-inflammatory properties, which can soothe the gut lining.

- o **Ingredients:** Turmeric powder, ginger, cinnamon, black pepper, water, honey (optional).

- o **How to Prepare:** Boil water with turmeric, ginger, cinnamon, and black pepper. Strain and add honey if desired.

- o **How to Use:** Drink warm.

- o **Dosage:** One cup daily.

- o **Side Effect:** May cause staining of clothes and utensils.

- o **Precaution:** Consult a doctor if you are on blood-thinning medications.

4. **Apple Cider Vinegar Tonic**

- o **Definition:** Supports healthy digestion and balances pH levels in the gut.

- o **Ingredients:** Apple cider vinegar, water, honey (optional).

- o **How to Prepare:** Mix apple cider vinegar with water. Add honey to taste.

- o **How to Use:** Consume before meals.

- o **Dosage:** One tablespoon diluted in a glass of water before each meal.

- o **Side Effect:** May erode tooth enamel if consumed undiluted.

- o **Precaution:** Dilute properly and use a straw to minimize contact with teeth.

5. Cabbage Juice Cleanse

- o **Definition:** Cabbage juice is rich in gut-friendly nutrients like glutamine and sulfur.

- o **Ingredients:** Fresh cabbage, water.

- o **How to Prepare:** Juice fresh cabbage using a juicer.

- o **How to Use:** Drink immediately after juicing.

- o **Dosage:** One glass daily.

- **Side Effect:** May cause flatulence in some individuals.

- **Precaution:** Start with a small amount to gauge tolerance.

6. Probiotic Yogurt Smoothie

- **Definition:** Provides beneficial probiotics to support a healthy gut microbiome.

- **Ingredients:** Plain yogurt, mixed berries, banana, honey (optional), almond milk.

- **How to Prepare:** Blend yogurt, mixed berries, banana, and almond milk until smooth.

- **How to Use:** Consume as a snack or breakfast option.

- **Dosage:** One serving per day.

- **Side Effect:** None expected, but individuals with lactose intolerance should use lactose-free yogurt.

- **Precaution:** Ensure yogurt contains live and active cultures.

7. Psyllium Husk Cleanse

- **Definition:** Psyllium husk is a soluble fiber that aids in bowel regularity and toxin removal.

- **Ingredients:** Psyllium husk powder, water.

- **How to Prepare:** Mix psyllium husk powder with water until fully dissolved.

- **How to Use:** Drink immediately followed by another glass of water.

- **Dosage:** Start with 1 teaspoon mixed in water, gradually increasing to 1 tablespoon daily.

- **Side Effect:** May cause bloating or gas initially.

- **Precaution:** Drink plenty of water to prevent choking risk.

8. Garlic and Honey Infusion

- **Definition:** Garlic has antimicrobial properties and honey soothes the digestive tract.

- **Ingredients:** Garlic cloves, honey.

- **How to Prepare:** Crush garlic cloves and mix with honey.

- **How to Use:** Consume a spoonful daily.

- **Dosage:** One teaspoon daily.

- **Side Effect:** Garlic may cause bad breath.

- **Precaution:** Avoid if allergic to garlic or honey.

9. Fermented Foods

- o **Definition:** Fermented foods like kimchi and sauerkraut contain probiotics that promote gut health.

- o **Ingredients:** Kimchi (cabbage, radish, garlic, chili peppers), sauerkraut (cabbage, salt).

- o **How to Prepare:** Purchase fermented foods from a trusted source or make them at home.

- o **How to Use:** Incorporate into meals as a side dish or snack.

- o **Dosage:** One serving daily.

- o **Side Effect:** May cause gas or bloating initially.

- o **Precaution:** Start with small servings to avoid digestive discomfort.

10. Dandelion Root Tea

- o **Definition:** Dandelion root supports liver function and aids digestion.

- o **Ingredients:** Dandelion root tea bags, water.

- o **How to Prepare:** Steep dandelion root tea bags in hot water for 5-10 minutes.

- o **How to Use:** Drink warm.

- **Dosage:** One cup daily.

- **Side Effect:** May cause allergic reactions in some individuals.

- **Precaution:** Consult a healthcare professional if pregnant or taking medications.

11. **Aloe Vera Juice Cleanse**

- **Definition:** Aloe vera juice can soothe and cleanse the digestive tract, aiding in detoxification.

- **Ingredients:** Fresh aloe vera gel, water, lemon juice (optional), honey (optional).

- **How to Prepare:** Blend fresh aloe vera gel with water and lemon juice. Add honey for sweetness if desired.

- **How to Use:** Drink on an empty stomach in the morning.

- **Dosage:** Start with a small amount (1-2 tablespoons) diluted in water, gradually increasing to 1/4 to 1/2 cup.

- **Side Effect:** May cause diarrhea or stomach cramps if consumed in excess.

- **Precaution:** Avoid if allergic to aloe vera or if experiencing abdominal pain.

12.   **Chia Seed Detox Water**

- o **Definition:** Chia seeds are rich in fiber and omega-3 fatty acids, promoting bowel regularity and gut health.

- o **Ingredients:** Chia seeds, water, lemon slices, mint leaves.

- o **How to Prepare:** Mix chia seeds with water and let it sit for 15-20 minutes until the seeds form a gel-like consistency. Add lemon slices and mint leaves for flavor.

- o **How to Use:** Drink throughout the day.

- o **Dosage:** One to two glasses daily.

- o **Side Effect:** May cause bloating if consumed without adequate water intake.

- o **Precaution:** Ensure chia seeds are well hydrated to prevent choking risk.

13.   **Ginger-Turmeric Shot**

- o **Definition:** Combines the anti-inflammatory properties of ginger and turmeric for gut health and immune support.

- o **Ingredients:** Fresh ginger, fresh turmeric, lemon juice, black pepper.

- o **How to Prepare:** Juice ginger and turmeric, then mix with lemon juice and a pinch of black pepper.

- o **How to Use:** Consume as a shot.

- o **Dosage:** One shot daily.

- o **Side Effect:** May cause heartburn in some individuals.

- o **Precaution:** Start with a small amount if sensitive to spicy foods.

14. **Papaya Seed Smoothie**

- o **Definition:** Papaya seeds contain enzymes that aid digestion and support the removal of parasites.

- o **Ingredients:** Papaya seeds, papaya chunks, pineapple, coconut water.

- o **How to Prepare:** Blend papaya seeds, papaya chunks, pineapple, and coconut water until smooth.

- o **How to Use:** Consume as a breakfast or snack option.

- o **Dosage:** One serving per day.

- o **Side Effect:** May cause a laxative effect if consumed in excess.

- o **Precaution:** Avoid if pregnant or breastfeeding.

15. **Activated Charcoal Detox Drink**

- o **Definition:** Activated charcoal binds to toxins in the gut, aiding in their removal from the body.

- o **Ingredients:** Activated charcoal powder, water, lemon juice, honey (optional).

- o **How to Prepare:** Mix activated charcoal powder with water, lemon juice, and honey.

- o **How to Use:** Drink on an empty stomach.

- o **Dosage:** Start with 1/2 teaspoon mixed in water, gradually increasing to 1 teaspoon.

- o **Side Effect:** May interfere with medication absorption if taken simultaneously.

- o **Precaution:** Take activated charcoal separately from medications and supplements.

CHAPTER NINE

Detoxification and Elimination: How Dr. Barbara's Protocol Supports the Body's Natural Cleansing Processes

Dr. Barbara's protocol for gut health and cleansing is designed to support the body's natural detoxification and elimination processes. By incorporating specific dietary strategies, herbal supplements, and lifestyle modifications, the protocol aims to optimize liver function, enhance toxin elimination, and promote overall well-being. Let's explore how Dr. Barbara's protocol supports detoxification and elimination:

1. Liver Support:

The liver plays a central role in detoxification, metabolizing toxins and facilitating their excretion from the body. Dr. Barbara's protocol includes herbs and nutrients that support liver function, such as:

- **Milk Thistle (Silybum marianum):** Milk thistle contains a compound called silymarin, which has antioxidant and anti-inflammatory properties that support liver health. It helps protect liver cells from damage and promotes detoxification.

- **Dandelion Root (Taraxacum officinale):** Dandelion root is a natural diuretic and liver tonic that supports liver function and promotes bile production, aiding in the elimination of toxins from the body.

- **Turmeric (Curcuma longa):** Turmeric contains the active compound curcumin, which has potent anti-inflammatory and antioxidant properties. It supports liver detoxification pathways and helps reduce oxidative stress.

2. Enhanced Digestive Function:

Optimal digestive function is essential for effective toxin elimination. Dr. Barbara's protocol includes herbs and nutrients that support digestion and promote regular bowel movements, such as:

- **Psyllium Husk:** Psyllium husk is a soluble fiber that absorbs water in the digestive tract, bulking up stool and promoting bowel regularity. It helps sweep toxins out of the intestines and supports detoxification.

- **Aloe Vera:** Aloe vera contains compounds called anthraquinones, which have laxative effects and promote bowel movements. It helps cleanse the colon and eliminate waste from the body.

- **Probiotics:** Beneficial bacteria found in probiotic supplements support gut health and promote the balance of intestinal flora. They aid in digestion, nutrient absorption, and the elimination of toxins from the body.

3. Antioxidant Support:

Antioxidants play a crucial role in neutralizing free radicals and reducing oxidative stress, which can damage cells and contribute to toxin buildup in the body. Dr. Barbara's protocol includes antioxidant-rich foods and supplements, such as:

- **Berries:** Berries are rich in antioxidants such as anthocyanins, flavonoids, and vitamin C, which help protect cells from oxidative damage and support detoxification.

- **Vitamin C:** As a powerful antioxidant, vitamin C helps neutralize free radicals and enhance the body's natural detoxification processes. It supports liver function and promotes the production of glutathione, a key antioxidant in detoxification.

- **Green Tea:** Green tea contains catechins, potent antioxidants that support liver health and promote detoxification. Drinking green tea regularly can help protect against toxin-induced liver damage.

4. Hydration and Elimination:

Proper hydration is essential for supporting detoxification and elimination processes. Dr. Barbara's protocol emphasizes the importance of staying hydrated and includes recommendations for increasing water intake, herbal teas, and hydrating foods such as fruits and vegetables.

- **Water:** Drinking an adequate amount of water throughout the day helps flush toxins from the body, support kidney function, and maintain overall hydration.

- **Herbal Teas:** Certain herbal teas, such as dandelion root tea, ginger tea, and peppermint tea, have diuretic and digestive properties that support detoxification and elimination.

- **Hydrating Foods:** Fruits and vegetables with high water content, such as cucumbers, watermelon, and celery, help hydrate the body and support detoxification by providing essential nutrients and fiber.

Conclusion:

Dr. Barbara's protocol for gut health and cleansing is designed to support the body's natural detoxification and elimination processes through targeted dietary strategies, herbal supplements, and lifestyle modifications. By incorporating liver-supportive herbs, digestive aids, antioxidants, and hydration recommendations, the protocol aims to optimize detoxification pathways, enhance toxin elimination, and promote overall well-being. Always consult with a healthcare professional before starting any new detoxification program, especially if you have underlying health conditions or are taking medications.

CHAPTER TEN

Post-Cleanse Maintenance: Strategies for Sustaining Gut Health Through Long-Term Dietary and Lifestyle Changes

Completing a gut cleanse is an empowering step towards improved digestive health, but sustaining these benefits requires ongoing commitment to long-term dietary and lifestyle changes. Post-cleanse maintenance involves implementing strategies that support gut health, promote microbial diversity, and prevent the recurrence of digestive issues. Here are some key strategies for sustaining gut health through long-term dietary and lifestyle changes:

1. Adopt a Gut-Friendly Diet:

- **Emphasize Whole, Plant-Based Foods:** Base your diet around whole, unprocessed plant foods such as fruits, vegetables, whole grains, legumes, nuts, and seeds. These foods are rich in fiber, antioxidants, vitamins, and minerals that support gut health and promote microbial diversity.

- **Include Fermented Foods:** Incorporate fermented foods such as yogurt, kefir, sauerkraut, kimchi, and kombucha into your diet. These foods are rich in beneficial probiotics that support a healthy gut microbiome and aid in digestion.

- **Limit Processed Foods and Sugars:** Minimize your intake of processed foods, refined sugars, artificial additives, and unhealthy fats, as these can disrupt gut health and contribute to inflammation and dysbiosis.

2. Prioritize Gut-Healthy Lifestyle Habits:

- **Stay Hydrated:** Drink plenty of water throughout the day to support hydration and promote healthy digestion. Aim for at least 8-10 glasses of water per day, and hydrate with herbal teas, coconut water, and infused water for added flavor.

- **Manage Stress:** Practice stress-reducing techniques such as meditation, deep breathing, yoga, tai chi, or mindfulness to support gut health and overall well-being. Chronic stress can disrupt digestion and contribute to gut issues, so prioritizing stress management is essential.

- **Get Regular Exercise:** Engage in regular physical activity to support digestion, promote bowel regularity, and maintain a healthy weight. Aim for a combination of cardiovascular exercise, strength training, and flexibility exercises for optimal health.

3. Support Digestive Function with Supplements:

- **Probiotics:** Consider taking a high-quality probiotic supplement to support gut health and maintain microbial balance. Look for a probiotic with a diverse range of bacterial strains and a high colony-forming unit (CFU) count.

- **Digestive Enzymes:** If you have difficulty digesting certain foods, consider taking digestive enzyme supplements to support digestion and nutrient absorption. Choose a broad-spectrum enzyme formula that includes enzymes for protein, fat, and carbohydrate digestion.

- **Fiber Supplements:** If you struggle to meet your fiber needs through diet alone, consider taking a fiber supplement to support digestive health and promote regular bowel movements. Look for a soluble fiber supplement such as psyllium husk or acacia fiber.

4. Practice Mindful Eating:

- **Eat Slowly and Mindfully:** Take time to chew your food thoroughly and savor each bite. Eating slowly and mindfully can help reduce overeating, improve digestion, and enhance nutrient absorption.

- **Listen to Your Body:** Pay attention to your body's hunger and fullness cues, and eat only when you're hungry. Avoid eating out of boredom, stress, or habit, and stop eating when you're comfortably satisfied.

5. Regularly Assess and Adjust Your Diet and Lifestyle:

- **Keep a Food Diary:** Track your dietary intake, symptoms, and overall well-being in a food diary to identify patterns and triggers. This can help you pinpoint foods that may be causing digestive issues and make informed decisions about your diet.

- **Be Flexible and Open-Minded:** Recognize that everyone's digestive system is unique, and what works for one person may not work for another. Stay open-minded and be willing to experiment with different foods, supplements, and lifestyle practices to find what works best for you.

Conclusion:

Sustaining gut health through long-term dietary and lifestyle changes requires ongoing commitment, but the benefits are well worth the effort. By adopting a gut-friendly diet, prioritizing gut-healthy lifestyle habits, supporting digestive function with supplements, practicing mindful eating, and regularly assessing and adjusting your diet and lifestyle, you can maintain optimal gut health and enjoy lasting improvements in digestion and overall well-being. Remember that consistency is key, and small, gradual changes can lead to significant long-term benefits for your gut health.

BONUS: SOME ESSENTIAL HERBAL REMEDIES FOR HEALTH AND WELLNESS

Cocolmeca:

Definition: Cocolmeca, also known as Smilax ornata or sarsaparilla, is a flowering vine native to Mexico and Central America. It has been used traditionally in Mexican and Central American folk medicine for its purported medicinal properties.

Ingredients: Cocolmeca contains various bioactive compounds, including saponins, flavonoids, and plant sterols. These compounds are believed to contribute to the herb's medicinal properties, including its potential as a diuretic, blood purifier, and anti-inflammatory agent.

How to Prepare: Cocolmeca is commonly prepared and consumed as an herbal tea or decoction. To make tea, dried cocolmeca roots or leaves are steeped in hot water for several minutes before being strained and consumed. Decoctions involve boiling the roots or leaves in water to extract their active compounds.

Dosage: The appropriate dosage of cocolmeca can vary depending on factors such as age, health status, and the specific preparation being used. It's important to follow the recommended dosage on the product label or consult with a qualified herbalist or healthcare professional for personalized guidance.

How to Use: Cocolmeca tea or decoction is typically taken orally. It can also be used topically for certain skin conditions. It's important to use cocolmeca products as directed and to discontinue use if any adverse effects occur.

Side Effects: Cocolmeca is generally considered safe for most people when used in moderate amounts. However, excessive intake may lead to digestive upset or other adverse effects. It may also interact with certain medications or have adverse effects in individuals with certain health conditions. It's important to use cocolmeca under the guidance of a healthcare professional and to discontinue use if any adverse effects occur.

Contribo:

Definition: Contribo, also known as Aristolochiatrilobata, is a vine native to the Caribbean and Central America. It has been used traditionally in folk medicine for various purposes, including as a remedy for digestive issues, inflammation, and pain relief.

Ingredients: Contribo contains several bioactive compounds, including aristolochic acids, flavonoids, and alkaloids. These compounds are believed to contribute to the herb's medicinal properties, including its potential as an anti-inflammatory and analgesic agent.

How to Prepare: Contribo is typically prepared and consumed as an herbal tea or decoction. To make tea, dried contribo leaves or stems are steeped in hot water for several minutes before being strained and consumed. Decoctions involve boiling the leaves or stems in water to extract their active compounds.

Dosage: The appropriate dosage of contribo can vary depending on factors such as age, health status, and the specific preparation being used. It's important to follow the recommended dosage on the product label or consult with a qualified herbalist or healthcare professional for personalized guidance.

How to Use: Contribo tea or decoction is typically taken orally. It's important to use contribo products as directed and to discontinue use if any adverse effects occur.

Side Effects: Contribo contains aristolochic acids, which have been associated with serious adverse effects, including kidney damage and cancer. Due to these safety concerns, the use of contribo is highly discouraged, and it's important to avoid products containing aristolochic acids. Individuals should seek alternative remedies for their health needs.

Dandelion Root:

Definition: Dandelion, scientifically known as Taraxacum officinale, is a common flowering plant found worldwide. While often considered a pesky weed, dandelion has a long history of use in traditional medicine for its various health benefits.

Ingredients: Dandelion root contains several bioactive compounds, including sesquiterpene lactones, triterpenes, flavonoids, and polysaccharides. These compounds are believed to contribute to the herb's medicinal properties, including its potential as a diuretic, digestive aid, and liver tonic.

How to Prepare: Dandelion root can be prepared and consumed in various forms, including teas, tinctures, capsules, and extracts. To make tea, dried dandelion root is steeped in hot water for several minutes before being strained and consumed. Tinctures are prepared by steeping the root in alcohol or vinegar to extract its active compounds.

Dosage: The appropriate dosage of dandelion root can vary depending on factors such as age, health status, and the specific preparation being used. It's important to follow the recommended dosage on the product label or consult with a qualified herbalist or healthcare professional for personalized guidance.

How to Use: Dandelion root tea, tincture, or capsules are typically taken orally. It's important to use dandelion root products as directed and to discontinue use if any adverse effects occur.

Side Effects: Dandelion root is generally considered safe for most people when used in moderate amounts. However, some individuals may experience allergic reactions or digestive upset. It may also interact with certain medications or have adverse effects in individuals with certain health conditions. It's important to use dandelion root under the guidance of a healthcare professional and to discontinue use if any adverse effects occur.

Green Food Plus:

Definition: Green Food Plus is a dietary supplement formulated to provide a concentrated source of nutrients derived from various green plants. It's designed to support overall health and well-being by delivering essential vitamins, minerals, antioxidants, and phytonutrients.

Ingredients: Green Food Plus typically contains a blend of powdered green vegetables, grasses, algae, and other plant-based ingredients. Common ingredients may include wheatgrass, barley grass, spirulina, chlorella, alfalfa, kale, spinach, and broccoli, among others.

How to Prepare: Green Food Plus is usually available in powder form and can be mixed with water, juice, or smoothies. It's important to follow the recommended dosage on the product label and to consume it as part of a balanced diet.

Dosage: The appropriate dosage of Green Food Plus can vary depending on the specific product and individual needs. It's important to follow the recommended dosage on the product label or consult with a healthcare professional for personalized guidance.

How to Use: Green Food Plus powder is typically mixed with water, juice, or smoothies and consumed orally. It's often taken once or twice daily, preferably with meals, to maximize nutrient absorption.

Side Effects: Green Food Plus is generally considered safe for most people when used as directed. However, some individuals may experience digestive upset or allergic reactions to certain ingredients. It's important to consult with a healthcare provider before starting any new supplement regimen, especially if you have underlying health conditions or are taking medications.

Hydrangea:

Definition: Hydrangea, scientifically known as Hydrangea arborescens, is a flowering shrub native to North America. It has been used traditionally in herbal medicine for its potential diuretic and anti-inflammatory properties.

Ingredients: Hydrangea contains several bioactive compounds, including saponins, flavonoids, and glycosides. These compounds are believed to contribute to the herb's medicinal properties, including its potential as a diuretic, kidney tonic, and anti-inflammatory agent.

How to Prepare: Hydrangea root is typically prepared and consumed as an herbal tea or tincture. To make tea, dried hydrangea root is steeped in hot water for several minutes before being strained and consumed. Tinctures are prepared by steeping the root in alcohol or vinegar to extract its active compounds.

Dosage: The appropriate dosage of hydrangea can vary depending on factors such as age, health status, and the specific preparation being used. It's important to follow the recommended dosage on the product label or consult with a qualified herbalist or healthcare professional for personalized guidance.

How to Use: Hydrangea tea or tincture is typically taken orally. It's important to use hydrangea products as directed and to discontinue use if any adverse effects occur.

Side Effects: Hydrangea is generally considered safe for most people when used in moderate amounts. However, some individuals may experience digestive upset or allergic reactions. It may also interact with certain medications or have adverse effects in individuals with certain health conditions. It's important to use hydrangea under the guidance of a healthcare professional and to discontinue use if any adverse effects occur.

Irish Moss:

Definition: Irish Moss, scientifically known as Chondrus crispus, is a species of red algae or seaweed native to the Atlantic coastlines of Europe and North America. It has been used for centuries in traditional Irish and Scottish cuisine, as well as in herbal medicine.

Ingredients: Irish Moss is rich in various nutrients, including iodine, sulfur compounds, vitamins (such as vitamin A, vitamin K, and vitamin B12), minerals (including calcium, magnesium, potassium, and sodium), and polysaccharides (such as carrageenan). These nutrients are believed to contribute to the herb's potential health benefits.

How to Prepare: Irish Moss is typically prepared by soaking it in water to rehydrate and soften it before use. It can be added to soups, stews, smoothies, desserts, and other dishes as a thickening agent or nutritional supplement.

Dosage: The appropriate dosage of Irish Moss can vary depending on factors such as age, health status, and the specific preparation being used. It's important to follow recipes or guidelines for culinary use and to consult with a healthcare professional for guidance on using Irish Moss as a dietary supplement.

How to Use: Irish Moss can be used in culinary applications to add thickness and nutritional value to dishes. It can also be consumed as a dietary supplement in the form of capsules, powders, or extracts.

Side Effects: Irish Moss is generally considered safe for most people when consumed in moderate amounts as part of a balanced diet. However, some individuals may be allergic to seaweed or carrageenan, a compound found in Irish Moss that is used as a food additive. It's important to discontinue use if any adverse effects occur and to consult with a healthcare professional if you have any concerns.

Irish Sea Moss:

Definition: Irish Sea Moss is a term often used interchangeably with Irish Moss, referring to the same species of red algae, Chondrus crispus. It's harvested from the rocky shores of the Atlantic coastlines of Europe and North America.

Ingredients: Irish Sea Moss shares the same nutritional profile as Irish Moss, containing iodine, vitamins, minerals, and polysaccharides. It's valued for its potential health benefits, including supporting thyroid function, boosting immune health, and promoting digestion.

How to Prepare: Irish Sea Moss is prepared in the same way as Irish Moss, by soaking it in water to rehydrate and soften it before use. It can be used in culinary applications or consumed as a dietary supplement.

Dosage: The dosage of Irish Sea Moss depends on the form and intended use. As a dietary supplement, it's important to follow the recommended dosage on the product label or consult with a healthcare professional for personalized guidance.

How to Use: Irish Sea Moss can be used in various culinary applications, including soups, smoothies, desserts, and sauces. It can also be consumed as a dietary supplement in the form of capsules, powders, or extracts.

Side Effects: Similar to Irish Moss, Irish Sea Moss is generally considered safe for most people when consumed in moderate amounts. However, individuals with seaweed allergies or sensitivities to carrageenan should exercise caution. It's important to discontinue use if any adverse effects occur and to consult with a healthcare professional if you have any concerns.

Lymphalin:

Definition: Lymphalin is a herbal supplement formulated to support lymphatic system health. The lymphatic system plays a crucial role in immune function and waste removal in the body, and Lymphalin is designed to promote its proper function.

Ingredients: Lymphalin typically contains a blend of herbs and botanical extracts known for their traditional use in supporting lymphatic system health. Common ingredients may include cleavers, red clover, echinacea, burdock root, and calendula, among others.

How to Prepare: Lymphalin is usually available in capsule or liquid form. Capsules are taken orally with water, while liquid forms may be mixed with water or juice before consumption. It's important to follow the recommended dosage on the product label.

Dosage: The appropriate dosage of Lymphalin can vary depending on the specific product and individual needs. It's important to follow the recommended dosage on the product label or consult with a healthcare professional for personalized guidance.

How to Use: Lymphalin capsules are typically taken orally with water, while liquid forms may be mixed with water or juice before consumption. It's often recommended to take Lymphalin on an empty stomach for optimal absorption.

Side Effects: Lymphalin is generally considered safe for most people when used as directed. However, some individuals may experience mild side effects such as gastrointestinal discomfort or allergic reactions to certain ingredients. It's important to consult with a healthcare provider before starting any new supplement regimen, especially if you have underlying health conditions or are taking medications.

Manjakani:

Definition: Manjakani, also known as Quercus infectoria or oak gall, is a natural substance derived from the oak tree. It has been used for centuries in traditional medicine for its potential health benefits, particularly for women's health and vaginal tightening.

Ingredients: Manjakani contains various bioactive compounds, including tannins, flavonoids, and gallic acid. These compounds are believed to contribute to the herb's medicinal properties, including its potential as an astringent and antiseptic agent.

How to Prepare: Manjakani is typically available in powder, capsule, or liquid extract form. It can be taken orally or used topically depending on the intended use. For vaginal tightening, manjakani may be applied topically as a gel or inserted into the vagina in capsule form.

Dosage: The appropriate dosage of manjakani can vary depending on factors such as age, health status, and the specific preparation being used. It's important to follow the recommended dosage on the product label or consult with a qualified herbalist or healthcare professional for personalized guidance.

How to Use: Manjakani can be taken orally or used topically depending on the intended use. It's important to use manjakani products as directed and to discontinue use if any adverse effects occur.

Side Effects: Manjakani is generally considered safe for most people when used in moderate amounts. However, some individuals may experience allergic reactions or skin irritation when used topically. It's important to use manjakani under the guidance of a healthcare professional and to discontinue use if any adverse effects occur.

Red Clover:

Definition: Red clover, scientifically known as Trifolium pratense, is a flowering plant belonging to the legume family. It's native to Europe, Western Asia, and Northwest Africa but has been naturalized in many other regions. Red clover has been used in traditional medicine for various purposes, including its potential to support women's health and menopausal symptoms.

Ingredients: Red clover contains several bioactive compounds, including isoflavones (such as genistein and daidzein), flavonoids, and phytoestrogens. These compounds are believed to contribute to the herb's medicinal properties, including its potential as a hormone-balancing agent and its ability to support cardiovascular health.

How to Prepare: Red clover is typically prepared and consumed as an herbal tea or tincture. To make tea, dried red clover flowers are steeped in hot water for several minutes before being strained and consumed. Tinctures are prepared by steeping the flowers in alcohol or vinegar to extract their active compounds.

Dosage: The appropriate dosage of red clover can vary depending on factors such as age, health status, and the specific preparation being used. It's important to follow the recommended dosage on the product label or consult with a qualified herbalist or healthcare professional for personalized guidance.

How to Use: Red clover tea or tincture is typically taken orally. It's important to use red clover products as directed and to discontinue use if any adverse effects occur.

Side Effects: Red clover is generally considered safe for most people when used in moderate amounts. However, some individuals may experience allergic reactions or digestive upset. It may also interact with certain medications or have adverse effects in individuals with certain health conditions. It's important to use red clover under the guidance of a healthcare professional and to discontinue use if any adverse effects occur.

Red Raspberry:

Definition: Red raspberry, scientifically known as Rubus idaeus, is a species of raspberry native to Europe and northern Asia. It's widely cultivated for its delicious berries and has been used in traditional medicine for various purposes, including its potential to support women's health during pregnancy and childbirth.

Ingredients: Red raspberry contains several bioactive compounds, including flavonoids, ellagic acid, anthocyanins, and vitamin C. These compounds are believed to contribute to the herb's medicinal properties, including its potential as an antioxidant, anti-inflammatory, and uterine tonic.

How to Prepare: Red raspberry leaf is typically prepared and consumed as an herbal tea or infusion. To make tea, dried red raspberry leaves are steeped in hot water for several minutes before being strained and consumed.

Dosage: The appropriate dosage of red raspberry leaf can vary depending on factors such as age, health status, and the specific preparation being used. It's important to follow the recommended dosage on the product label or consult with a qualified herbalist or healthcare professional for personalized guidance.

How to Use: Red raspberry leaf tea is typically taken orally. It's often recommended for pregnant individuals in the later stages of pregnancy to support uterine health and prepare for childbirth. It's important to use red raspberry leaf products as directed and to discontinue use if any adverse effects occur.

Side Effects: Red raspberry leaf is generally considered safe for most people when used in moderate amounts. However, some individuals may experience allergic reactions or digestive upset. Pregnant individuals should consult with a healthcare professional before using red raspberry leaf, especially if they have any underlying health conditions or are taking medications. It's important to use red raspberry leaf under the guidance of a healthcare professional and to discontinue use if any adverse effects occur.

Rhubarb:

Definition: Rhubarb, scientifically known as Rheum rhabarbarum, is a perennial plant cultivated for its edible stalks. While primarily used in culinary applications, rhubarb has also been utilized in traditional medicine for its potential health benefits, particularly for digestive health.

Ingredients: Rhubarb stalks contain various bioactive compounds, including anthraquinones (such as emodin and rhein), fiber, vitamins (such as vitamin K), and minerals (including calcium and potassium). These compounds are believed to contribute to the herb's medicinal properties, including its potential as a laxative and digestive aid.

How to Prepare: Rhubarb stalks are typically cooked before consumption, as the raw stalks are very tart and can be unpleasant to eat. They are often used in pies, crisps, jams, sauces, and other desserts, as well as in savory dishes. Rhubarb can also be used to make compotes, jams, and preserves.

Dosage: There is no specific dosage for rhubarb in culinary applications, as it is used as a food rather than a medicinal herb. However, when used for its potential laxative effects, it's important to consume rhubarb in moderation to avoid gastrointestinal upset.

How to Use: Rhubarb stalks can be chopped and cooked in various dishes, including pies, sauces, and jams. It's important to remove and discard the leaves, as they contain toxic compounds.

When using rhubarb for its potential laxative effects, it's typically consumed as part of a cooked dish or in the form of a rhubarb-based herbal remedy.

Side Effects: Rhubarb stalks are generally safe for most people when consumed in moderate amounts as part of a balanced diet. However, excessive intake may lead to digestive upset or adverse effects due to the presence of oxalic acid, which can bind to calcium and form kidney stones in susceptible individuals. It's important to use rhubarb in moderation and to consult with a healthcare professional if you have any concerns or underlying health conditions.

Sarsaparilla:

Definition: Sarsaparilla refers to several species of plants belonging to the Smilax genus, including Smilax regelii and Smilax officinalis. It has been used historically in traditional medicine for its potential health benefits, particularly for its purported detoxifying and anti-inflammatory properties.

Ingredients: Sarsaparilla contains various bioactive compounds, including saponins (such as sarsaponin and smilagenin), flavonoids, phenolic acids, and sterols. These compounds are believed to contribute to the herb's medicinal properties, including its potential as a diuretic, blood purifier, and anti-inflammatory agent.

How to Prepare: Sarsaparilla root is typically prepared and consumed as an herbal tea, decoction, or tincture. To make tea, dried sarsaparilla root is steeped in hot water for several minutes before being strained and consumed. Decoctions involve boiling the root in water to extract its active compounds, while tinctures are prepared by steeping the root in alcohol or vinegar.

Dosage: The appropriate dosage of sarsaparilla can vary depending on factors such as age, health status, and the specific preparation being used. It's important to follow the recommended dosage on the product label or consult with a qualified herbalist or healthcare professional for personalized guidance.

How to Use: Sarsaparilla tea or tincture is typically taken orally. It's important to use sarsaparilla products as directed and to discontinue use if any adverse effects occur.

Side Effects: Sarsaparilla is generally considered safe for most people when used in moderate amounts. However, some individuals may experience allergic reactions or digestive upset. It may also interact with certain medications or have adverse effects in individuals with certain health conditions. It's important to use sarsaparilla under the guidance of a healthcare professional and to discontinue use if any adverse effects occur.

Tila:

Definition: Tila, also known as linden flower or lime blossom, refers to the flowers of the Tilia genus, primarily Tilia europaea and Tilia cordata. These trees are native to Europe, but they are also cultivated in other regions for their fragrant and medicinal flowers.

Ingredients: Tila flowers contain various bioactive compounds, including flavonoids, phenolic acids, and volatile oils. These compounds are believed to contribute to the herb's medicinal properties, including its potential as a mild sedative, anxiolytic, and anti-inflammatory agent.

How to Prepare: Tila flowers are typically prepared and consumed as an herbal tea or infusion. To make tea, dried tila flowers are steeped in hot water for several minutes before being strained and consumed.

Dosage: The appropriate dosage of tila can vary depending on factors such as age, health status, and the specific preparation being used. It's important to follow the recommended dosage on the product label or consult with a qualified herbalist or healthcare professional for personalized guidance.

How to Use: Tila tea is typically taken orally. It's often consumed in the evening as a calming bedtime beverage or during times of stress or anxiety. It's important to use tila products as directed and to discontinue use if any adverse effects occur.

Side Effects: Tila is generally considered safe for most people when used in moderate amounts. However, some individuals may experience allergic reactions or digestive upset. It may also interact with certain medications or have adverse effects in individuals with certain health conditions. It's important to use tila under the guidance of a healthcare professional and to discontinue use if any adverse effects occur.

Valerian:

Definition: Valerian, scientifically known as Valeriana officinalis, is a perennial flowering plant native to Europe and Asia. It has been used for centuries in traditional medicine for its potential calming and sedative effects.

Ingredients: Valerian root contains several bioactive compounds, including valerenic acid, valepotriates, and volatile oils. These compounds are believed to contribute to the herb's medicinal properties, including its potential as a sedative, anxiolytic, and sleep aid.

How to Prepare: Valerian root is typically prepared and consumed as an herbal tea, tincture, or capsule. To make tea, dried valerian root is steeped in hot water for several minutes before being strained and consumed. Tinctures are prepared by steeping the root in alcohol or vinegar to extract its active compounds.

Dosage: The appropriate dosage of valerian can vary depending on factors such as age, health status, and the specific preparation being used. It's important to follow the recommended dosage on the product label or consult with a qualified herbalist or healthcare professional for personalized guidance.

How to Use: Valerian tea, tincture, or capsules are typically taken orally. It's often consumed in the evening as a sleep aid or during times of stress or anxiety. It's important to use valerian products as directed and to discontinue use if any adverse effects occur.

Side Effects: Valerian is generally considered safe for most people when used in moderate amounts. However, some individuals may experience mild side effects such as drowsiness, headache, or gastrointestinal upset. It may also interact with certain medications or have adverse effects in individuals with certain health conditions. It's important to use valerian under the guidance of a healthcare professional and to discontinue use if any adverse effects occur.

Wild Cherry Bark:

Definition: Wild cherry bark, scientifically known as Prunus serotina, is the bark obtained from the black cherry tree native to North America. It has been used traditionally in Native American and folk medicine for its potential health benefits, particularly for respiratory and digestive issues.

Ingredients: Wild cherry bark contains various bioactive compounds, including cyanogenic glycosides (such as prunasin and amygdalin), flavonoids, and phenolic acids. These compounds are believed to contribute to the herb's medicinal properties, including its potential as an expectorant, cough suppressant, and mild sedative.

How to Prepare: Wild cherry bark is typically prepared and consumed as an herbal tea, decoction, or syrup. To make tea, dried wild cherry bark is steeped in hot water for several minutes before being strained and consumed. Decoctions involve boiling the bark in water to extract its active compounds, while syrups are made by simmering the bark with sugar or honey to create a thick, sweet liquid.

Dosage: The appropriate dosage of wild cherry bark can vary depending on factors such as age, health status, and the specific preparation being used. It's important to follow the recommended dosage on the product label or consult with a qualified herbalist or healthcare professional for personalized guidance.

How to Use: Wild cherry bark tea, decoction, or syrup is typically taken orally. It's often consumed to soothe coughs, sore throats, and other respiratory symptoms. It's important to use wild cherry bark products as directed and to discontinue use if any adverse effects occur.

Side Effects: Wild cherry bark is generally considered safe for most people when used in moderate amounts. However, it contains cyanogenic glycosides, which can release cyanide in the body when metabolized. While the risk of cyanide poisoning from consuming wild cherry bark is low when used appropriately, excessive intake or prolonged use may lead to adverse effects. It's important to use wild cherry bark under the guidance of a healthcare professional and to discontinue use if any adverse effects occur.

Agrimony:

Definition: Agrimony, scientifically known as Agrimonia eupatoria, is a perennial herbaceous plant native to Europe, Asia, and North America. It has a long history of use in traditional medicine, particularly in European folk medicine, for its potential health benefits.

Ingredients: Agrimony contains various bioactive compounds, including tannins, flavonoids, phenolic acids, and volatile oils. These compounds are believed to contribute to the herb's medicinal properties, including its potential as an astringent, anti-inflammatory, and digestive aid.

How to Prepare: Agrimony is typically prepared and consumed as an herbal tea, tincture, or poultice. To make tea, dried agrimony leaves and flowers are steeped in hot water for several minutes before being strained and consumed. Tinctures are prepared by steeping the herb in alcohol or vinegar to extract its active compounds.

Dosage: The appropriate dosage of agrimony can vary depending on factors such as age, health status, and the specific preparation being used. It's important to follow the recommended dosage on the product label or consult with a qualified herbalist or healthcare professional for personalized guidance.

How to Use: Agrimony tea, tincture, or poultice is typically taken orally or applied topically. It's often consumed to soothe gastrointestinal issues, such as indigestion and diarrhea, or used externally to treat skin conditions.

Side Effects: Agrimony is generally considered safe for most people when used in moderate amounts. However, some individuals may experience allergic reactions or gastrointestinal upset. It may also interact with certain medications or have adverse effects in individuals with certain health conditions. It's important to use agrimony under the guidance of a healthcare professional and to discontinue use if any adverse effects occur.

Alfalfa:

Definition: Alfalfa, scientifically known as Medicago sativa, is a flowering plant in the pea family native to Asia but cultivated worldwide. It's primarily grown as fodder for livestock, but it has also been used in traditional medicine for its potential health benefits.

Ingredients: Alfalfa contains various bioactive compounds, including vitamins (such as vitamin A, vitamin C, and vitamin K), minerals (including calcium, magnesium, and potassium), amino acids, and phytoestrogens. These compounds are believed to contribute to the herb's medicinal properties, including its potential as a nutritive tonic, diuretic, and hormone balancer.

How to Prepare: Alfalfa is typically consumed as sprouts, herbal tea, or in supplement form (such as capsules or tablets). To make tea, dried alfalfa leaves are steeped in hot water for several minutes before being strained and consumed.

Dosage: The appropriate dosage of alfalfa can vary depending on factors such as age, health status, and the specific preparation being used. It's important to follow the recommended dosage on the product label or consult with a qualified herbalist or healthcare professional for personalized guidance.

How to Use: Alfalfa sprouts, tea, or supplements are typically taken orally. It's often consumed as a dietary supplement to support overall health and well-being, as well as to promote kidney health and hormone balance.

Side Effects: Alfalfa is generally considered safe for most people when consumed in moderate amounts. However, some individuals may experience allergic reactions or digestive upset. It may also interact with certain medications or have adverse effects in individuals with certain health conditions, such as autoimmune diseases or hormone-sensitive conditions. Pregnant or breastfeeding individuals should consult with a healthcare professional before using alfalfa supplements. It's important to use alfalfa under the guidance of a healthcare professional and to discontinue use if any adverse effects occur.

Yellowdock:

Definition: Yellowdock, scientifically known as Rumex crispus, is a perennial flowering plant native to Europe and western Asia but is also found in North America. It has a long history of use in traditional medicine, particularly among Indigenous peoples, for its potential health benefits.

Ingredients: Yellowdock root contains various bioactive compounds, including anthraquinone glycosides (such as emodin and chrysophanol), tannins, and vitamins (including vitamin A and vitamin C). These compounds are believed to contribute to the herb's medicinal properties, including its potential as a laxative, blood cleanser, and liver tonic.

How to Prepare: Yellowdock root is typically prepared and consumed as an herbal tea, tincture, or capsule. To make tea, dried yellowdock root is steeped in hot water for several minutes before being strained and consumed. Tinctures are prepared by steeping the root in alcohol or vinegar to extract its active compounds.

Dosage: The appropriate dosage of yellowdock can vary depending on factors such as age, health status, and the specific preparation being used. It's important to follow the recommended dosage on the product label or consult with a qualified herbalist or healthcare professional for personalized guidance.

How to Use: Yellowdock tea, tincture, or capsules are typically taken orally. It's often consumed to support digestion, promote bowel regularity, and cleanse the blood. It's important to use yellowdock products as directed and to discontinue use if any adverse effects occur.

Side Effects: Yellowdock is generally considered safe for most people when used in moderate amounts. However, some individuals may experience mild side effects such as gastrointestinal upset or allergic reactions. It may also interact with certain medications or have adverse effects in individuals with certain health conditions. It's important to use yellowdock under the guidance of a healthcare professional and to discontinue use if any adverse effects occur.

Yellowdock Root:

Definition: Yellowdock root, scientifically known as Rumex crispus, is the root of a perennial flowering plant native to Europe and western Asia, also found in North America. It has a long history of use in traditional medicine, particularly among Indigenous peoples, for its potential health benefits.

Ingredients: Yellowdock root contains various bioactive compounds, including anthraquinone glycosides (such as emodin and chrysophanol), tannins, and vitamins (including vitamin A and vitamin C). These compounds are believed to contribute to the herb's medicinal properties, including its potential as a laxative, blood cleanser, and liver tonic.

How to Prepare: Yellowdock root is typically prepared and consumed as an herbal tea, tincture, or capsule. To make tea, dried yellowdock root is steeped in hot water for several minutes before being strained and consumed. Tinctures are prepared by steeping the root in alcohol or vinegar to extract its active compounds.

Dosage: The appropriate dosage of yellowdock root can vary depending on factors such as age, health status, and the specific preparation being used. It's important to follow the recommended dosage on the product label or consult with a qualified herbalist or healthcare professional for personalized guidance.

How to Use: Yellowdock root tea, tincture, or capsules are typically taken orally. It's often consumed to support digestion, promote bowel regularity, and cleanse the blood. It's important to use yellowdock root products as directed and to discontinue use if any adverse effects occur.

Side Effects: Yellowdock root is generally considered safe for most people when used in moderate amounts. However, some individuals may experience mild side effects such as gastrointestinal upset or allergic reactions. It may also interact with certain medications or have adverse effects in individuals with certain health conditions. It's important to use yellowdock root under the guidance of a healthcare professional and to discontinue use if any adverse effects occur.

Guaco:

Definition: Guaco, also known as Mikania cordata or Mikania glomerata, is a medicinal plant native to Central and South America. It has a long history of use in traditional medicine for its potential therapeutic properties.

Ingredients: Guaco contains several bioactive compounds, including coumarins, flavonoids, tannins, and saponins. These compounds are believed to contribute to the herb's medicinal properties, including its potential as an expectorant, anti-inflammatory, and antispasmodic agent.

How to Prepare: Guaco is typically prepared and consumed as an herbal tea or infusion. To make tea, dried guaco leaves are steeped in hot water for several minutes before being strained and consumed.

Dosage: The appropriate dosage of guaco can vary depending on factors such as age, health status, and the specific preparation being used. It's important to follow the recommended dosage on the product label or consult with a qualified herbalist or healthcare professional for personalized guidance.

How to Use: Guaco tea is typically taken orally. It can be consumed on its own or mixed with honey or other herbal teas for added flavor.

Side Effects: Guaco is generally considered safe for most people when used in moderate amounts. However, some individuals may experience allergic reactions or digestive upset. It may also interact with certain medications or have adverse effects in individuals with certain health conditions. It's important to use guaco under the guidance of a healthcare professional and to discontinue use if any adverse effects occur.

Herban Iron:

Definition: Herban Iron is a dietary supplement designed to provide an easily absorbable form of iron to support healthy iron levels in the body. It's particularly beneficial for individuals with iron deficiency or anemia.

Ingredients: Herban Iron typically contains iron in the form of ferrous bisglycinate, which is a highly bioavailable and gentle form of iron that is less likely to cause digestive upset or constipation compared to other forms of iron. It may also contain other ingredients such as vitamin C to enhance iron absorption.

How to Prepare: Herban Iron is usually available in capsule or liquid form. Capsules are taken orally with water, while liquid forms may be mixed with water or juice before consumption. It's important to follow the recommended dosage on the product label.

Dosage: The appropriate dosage of Herban Iron depends on factors such as age, gender, and the severity of iron deficiency. It's important to consult with a healthcare professional to determine the correct dosage for individual needs.

How to Use: Herban Iron capsules are typically taken orally with water, while liquid forms may be mixed with water or juice before consumption. It's important to take Herban Iron as directed and to avoid taking it with dairy products, antacids, or other substances that may interfere with iron absorption.

Side Effects: While Herban Iron is generally considered safe for most people when used as directed, some individuals may experience mild side effects such as gastrointestinal discomfort or constipation. It's important to consult with a healthcare professional before starting any new supplement regimen, especially if you have underlying health conditions or are taking medications.

THE END

www.ingramcontent.com/pod-product-compliance
Lightning Source LLC
Chambersburg PA
CBHW081557250726
48653CB00009B/3475